My Diabetic Diet Cookbook

50 Amazing Meat, Seafood & Vegetable Diabetic Recipes

Valerie Blanchard

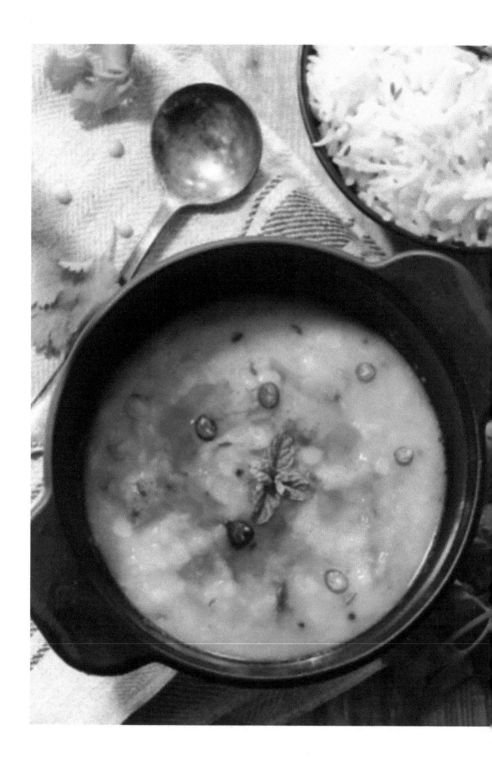

Table of Contents

6

Sesame Pork with Mustard Sauce

Preparation Time: 25 minutes

Cooking Time: 25 minutes

Servings: *4*

Ingredients:

- 2 tablespoons low-sodium teriyaki sauce
- ¼ cup chili sauce
- 2 cloves garlic, minced
- 2 teaspoons ginger, grated
- 2 pork tenderloins
- 2 teaspoons sesame seeds
- ¼ cup low fat sour cream
- 1 teaspoon Dijon mustard
- Salt to taste
- 1 scallion, chopped

Directions:

1. Preheat your oven to 425 degrees F.
2. Mix the teriyaki sauce, chili sauce, garlic and ginger.
3. Put the pork on a roasting pan.

4. Brush the sauce on both sides of the pork.

5. Bake in the oven for 15 minutes.

6. Brush with more sauce.

7. Top with sesame seeds.

8. Roast for 10 more minutes.

9. Mix the rest of the ingredients.

10. Serve the pork with mustard sauce.

Nutrition: Calories 135; Total Fat 3 g; Saturated Fat 1 g; Cholesterol 56 mg; Sodium 302 mg; Total Carbohydrate 7 g; Dietary Fiber 1 g; Total Sugars 15 g; Protein 20 g; Potassium 755 mg

Steak with Mushroom Sauce

Preparation Time: 20 minutes

Cooking Time: 5 minutes

Servings: *4*

Ingredients:

- 12 oz. sirloin steak, sliced and trimmed
- 2 teaspoons grilling seasoning
- 2 teaspoons oil
- 6 oz. broccoli, trimmed
- 2 cups frozen peas
- 3 cups fresh mushrooms, sliced
- 1 cup beef broth (unsalted)
- 1 tablespoon mustard
- 2 teaspoons cornstarch
- Salt to taste

Directions:

1. Preheat your oven to 350 degrees F.
2. Season meat with grilling seasoning.
3. In a pan over medium high heat, cook the meat and broccoli for 4 minutes.

4. Sprinkle the peas around the steak.

5. Put the pan inside the oven and bake for 8 minutes.

6. Remove both meat and vegetables from the pan.

7. Add the mushrooms to the pan.

8. Cook for 3 minutes.

9. Mix the broth, mustard, salt and cornstarch.

10. Add to the mushrooms.

11. Cook for 1 minute.

12. Pour sauce over meat and vegetables before serving.

Nutrition: Calories 226; Total Fat 6 g; Saturated Fat 2 g; Cholesterol 51 mg; Sodium 356 mg; Total Carbohydrate 16 g; Dietary Fiber 5 g; Total Sugars 6 g; Protein 26 g; Potassium 780 mg

Steak with Tomato & Herbs

Preparation Time: 30 minutes

Cooking Time: 30 minutes

Servings: *2*

Ingredients:

- 8 oz. beef loin steak, sliced in half
- Salt and pepper to taste
- Cooking spray
- 1 teaspoon fresh basil, snipped
- ¼ cup green onion, sliced
- 1/2 cup tomato, chopped

Directions:

1. Season the steak with salt and pepper.
2. Spray oil on your pan.
3. Put the pan over medium high heat.
4. Once hot, add the steaks.
5. Reduce heat to medium.
6. Cook for 10 to 13 minutes for medium, turning once.
7. Add the basil and green onion.
8. Cook for 2 minutes.

9. Add the tomato.

10. Cook for 1 minute.

11. Let cool a little before slicing.

Nutrition: Calories 170; Total Fat 6 g; Saturated Fat 2 g; Cholesterol 66 mg;Sodium 207 mg; Total Carbohydrate 3 g; Dietary Fiber 1 g; Total Sugars 5 g; Protein 25 g;Potassium 477 mg

Barbecue Beef Brisket

Preparation Time: 25 minutes

Cooking Time: *10 hours*

Servings: *10*

Ingredients:

- 4 lb. beef brisket (boneless), trimmed and sliced
- 1 bay leaf
- 2 onions, sliced into rings
- 1/2 teaspoon dried thyme, crushed
- ¼ cup chili sauce
- 1 clove garlic, minced
- Salt and pepper to taste
- 2 tablespoons light brown sugar
- 2 tablespoons cornstarch
- 2 tablespoons cold water

Directions:

1. Put the meat in a slow cooker.
2. Add the bay leaf and onion.

3. In a bowl, mix the thyme, chili sauce, salt, pepper and sugar.

4. Pour the sauce over the meat.

5. Mix well.

6. Seal the pot and cook on low heat for 10 hours.

7. Discard the bay leaf.

8. Pour cooking liquid in a pan.

9. Add the mixed water and cornstarch.

10. Simmer until the sauce has thickened.

11. Pour the sauce over the meat.

Nutrition: Calories 182; Total Fat 6 g;Saturated Fat 2 g; Cholesterol 57 mg; Sodium 217 mg; Total Sugars 4 g; Protein 20 g; Potassium 383 mg

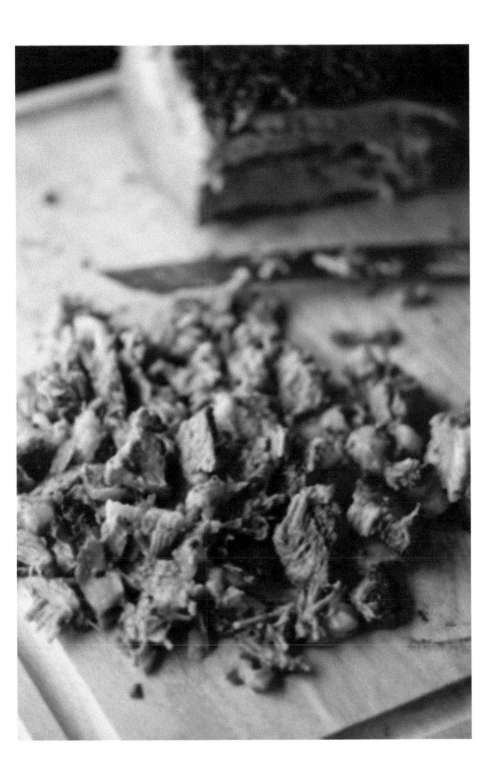

Beef & Asparagus

Preparation Time: 15 minutes

Cooking Time: 10 minutes

Servings: *4*

Ingredients:

- 2 teaspoons olive oil
- 1 lb. lean beef sirloin, trimmed and sliced
- 1 carrot, shredded
- Salt and pepper to taste
- 12 oz. asparagus, trimmed and sliced
- 1 teaspoon dried herbes de Provence, crushed
- 1/2 cup Marsala
- ¼ teaspoon lemon zest

Directions:

1. Pour oil in a pan over medium heat.
2. Add the beef and carrot.
3. Season with salt and pepper.
4. Cook for 3 minutes.
5. Add the asparagus and herbs.

6. Cook for 2 minutes.

7. Add the Marsala and lemon zest.

8. Cook for 5 minutes, stirring frequently.

Nutrition: Calories 327; Total Fat 7 g; Saturated Fat 2 g; Cholesterol 69 mg; Sodium 209 mg ;Total Carbohydrate 29 g; Dietary Fiber 2 g; Total Sugars 3 g; Protein 28 g; Potassium 576 mg

Italian Beef

Preparation Time: 20 minutes

Cooking Time: 1 hour and 20 minutes

Servings: *4*

Ingredients:

- Cooking spray
- 1 lb. beef round steak, trimmed and sliced
- 1 cup onion, chopped
- 2 cloves garlic, minced
- 1 cup green bell pepper, chopped
- 1/2 cup celery, chopped
- 2 cups mushrooms, sliced
- 14 1/2 oz. canned diced tomatoes
- 1/2 teaspoon dried basil
- ¼ teaspoon dried oregano
- 1/8 teaspoon crushed red pepper
- 2 tablespoons Parmesan cheese, grated

Directions:

1. Spray oil on the pan over medium heat.

2. Cook the meat until brown on both sides.

3. Transfer meat to a plate.

4. Add the onion, garlic, bell pepper, celery and mushroom to the pan.

5. Cook until tender.

6. Add the tomatoes, herbs, and pepper.

7. Put the meat back to the pan.

8. Simmer while covered for 1 hour and 15 minutes.

9. Stir occasionally.

10. Sprinkle Parmesan cheese on top of the dish before serving.

Nutrition: Calories 212; Total Fat 4 g; Saturated Fat 1 g; Cholesterol 51 mg; Sodium 296 mg; Total Sugars 6 g; Protein 30 g; Potassium 876 mg

Lamb with Broccoli & Carrots

Preparation Time: 20 minutes

Cooking Time: 10 minutes

Servings: *4*

Ingredients:

- 2 cloves garlic, minced
- 1 tablespoon fresh ginger, grated
- ¼ teaspoon red pepper, crushed
- 2 tablespoons low-sodium soy sauce
- 1 tablespoon white vinegar
- 1 tablespoon cornstarch
- 12 oz. lamb meat, trimmed and sliced
- 2 teaspoons cooking oil
- 1 lb. broccoli, sliced into florets
- 2 carrots, sliced into strips
- ¾ cup low-sodium beef broth
- 4 green onions, chopped
- 2 cups cooked spaghetti squash pasta

Directions:

1. Combine the garlic, ginger, red pepper, soy sauce, vinegar and cornstarch in a bowl.
2. Add lamb to the marinade.
3. Marinate for 10 minutes.
4. Discard marinade.
5. In a pan over medium heat, add the oil.
6. Add the lamb and cook for 3 minutes.
7. Transfer lamb to a plate.
8. Add the broccoli and carrots.
9. Cook for 1 minute.
10. Pour in the beef broth.
11. Cook for 5 minutes.
12. Put the meat back to the pan.
13. Sprinkle with green onion and serve on top of spaghetti squash.

Nutrition: Calories 205; Total Fat 6 g; Saturated Fat 1 g; Cholesterol 40 mg; Sodium 659 mg; Total Carbohydrate 17 g

Rosemary Lamb

Preparation Time: 15 minutes

Cooking Time: *2 hours*

Servings: *14*

Ingredients:

- Salt and pepper to taste
- 2 teaspoons fresh rosemary, snipped
- 5 lb. whole leg of lamb, trimmed and cut with slits on all sides
- 3 cloves garlic, slivered
- 1 cup water

Directions:

1. Preheat your oven to 375 degrees F.
2. Mix salt, pepper and rosemary in a bowl.
3. Sprinkle mixture all over the lamb.
4. Insert slivers of garlic into the slits.
5. Put the lamb on a roasting pan.
6. Add water to the pan.
7. Roast for 2 hours.

_Nutrition__:_ Calories 136; Total Fat 4 g; Saturated Fat 1 g; Cholesterol 71 mg; Sodium 218 mg; Protein 23 g; Potassium 248 mg

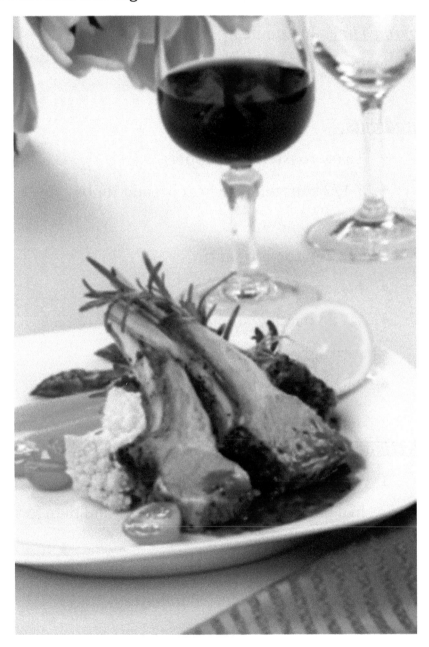

Mediterranean Lamb Meatballs

Preparation Time: 10 minutes

Cooking Time: 20 minutes

Servings: *8*

Ingredients:

- 12 oz. roasted red peppers
- 1 1/2 cups whole wheat breadcrumbs
- 2 eggs, beaten
- 1/3 cup tomato sauce
- 1/2 cup fresh basil
- ¼ cup parsley, snipped
- Salt and pepper to taste
- 2 lb. lean ground lamb

Directions:

1. Preheat your oven to 350 degrees F.
2. In a bowl, mix all the Ingredients and then form into meatballs.
3. Put the meatballs on a baking pan.
4. Bake in the oven for 20 minutes.

Nutrition: Calories 94; Total Fat 3 g; Saturated Fat 1 g; Cholesterol 35 mg; Sodium 170 mg; Total Carbohydrate 2 g; Dietary Fiber 1 g; Total Sugars 0 g

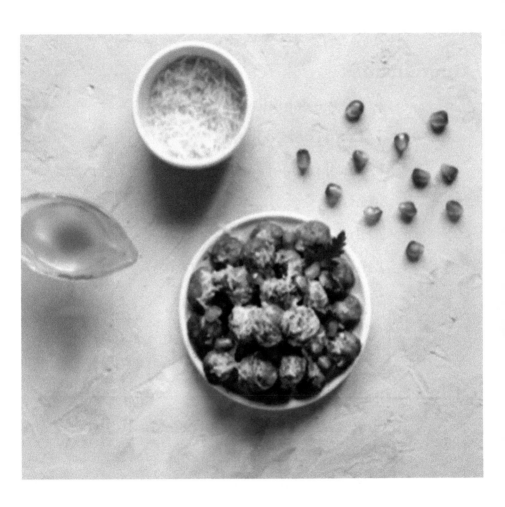

Cauliflower Rice with Chicken

Preparation Time: 15 Minutes

Cooking Time: 15 Minutes

Servings: *4*

Ingredients:

- 1/2 large cauliflower
- 3/4 cup cooked meat
- 1/2 bell pepper
- 1 carrot
- 2 ribs celery
- 1 tbsp. stir fry sauce (low carb)
- 1 tbsp. extra virgin olive oil
- Salt and pepper to taste

Directions:

1. Chop cauliflower in a processor to "rice." Place in a bowl.
2. Properly chop all vegetables in a food processor into thin slices.
3. Add cauliflower and other plants to WOK with heated oil. Fry until all veggies are tender.

4. Add chopped meat and sauce to the wok and fry 10 Minutes.
5. Serve

This dish is very mouth-watering!

__Nutrition:__ Calories 200; Protein 10 g; Fat 12 g; Carbs 10 g

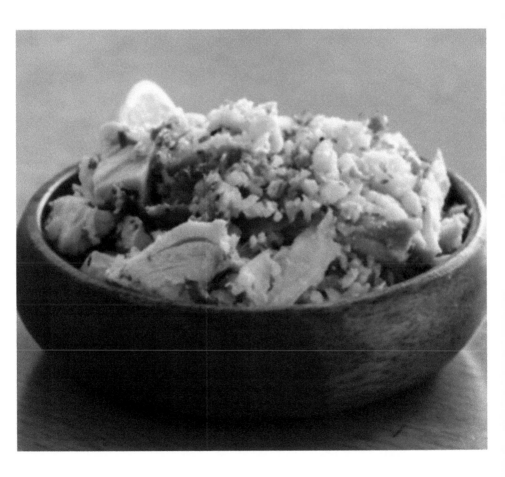

Turkey with Fried Eggs

__Preparation Time:__ 10 Minutes

Cooking Time*: 20 Minutes*
 Servings: *4*

Ingredients:

- 4 large potatoes
- 1 cooked turkey thigh
- 1 large onion (about 2 cups diced)
- butter
- Chile flakes
- 4 eggs
- salt to taste
- pepper to taste

__Directions:__

1. Rub the cold boiled potatoes on the coarsest holes of a box grater. Dice the turkey.

2. Cook the onion in as much unsalted butter as you feel comfortable with until it's just fragrant and translucent.

3. Add the rubbed potatoes and a cup of diced cooked turkey, salt and pepper to taste, and cook 20 Minutes.

Top each with a fried egg. Yummy!

Nutrition: Calories 170; Protein 19 g; Fat 7 g; Carbs 6 g

Sweet Potato, Kale, and White Bean Stew

Preparation Time: 15 minutes

Cooking Time: 25 minutes

Servings: *4*

Ingredients:

- 1 (15-ounce) can low-sodium cannellini beans, rinsed and drained, divided
- 1 tablespoon olive oil
- 1 medium onion, chopped
- 2 garlic cloves, minced
- 2 celery stalks, chopped
- 3 medium carrots, chopped
- 2 cups low-sodium vegetable broth
- 1 teaspoon apple cider vinegar
- 2 medium sweet potatoes (about 1¼ pounds)
- 2 cups chopped kale
- 1 cup shelled edamame
- ¼ cup quinoa
- 1 teaspoon dried thyme
- 1/2 teaspoon cayenne pepper
- 1/2 teaspoon salt

- ¼ teaspoon freshly ground black pepper

Directions:

1. Put half the beans into a blender and blend until smooth. Set aside.

2. In a large soup pot over medium heat, heat the oil. When the oil is shining, include the onion and garlic, and cook until the onion softens and the garlic is sweet, about 3 minutes. Add the celery and carrots, and continue cooking until the vegetables soften, about 5 minutes.

3. Add the broth, vinegar, sweet potatoes, unblended beans, kale, edamame, and quinoa, and bring the mixture to a boil. Reduce the heat and simmer until the vegetables soften, about 10 minutes.

4. Add the blended beans, thyme, cayenne, salt, and black pepper, increase the heat to medium-high, and bring the mixture to a boil. Reduce the heat and simmer, uncovered, until the flavors combine, about 5 minutes.

5. Into each of 4 containers, scoop 1¾ cups of stew.

Nutrition: Calories: 373; Total Fat: 7g; Saturated Fat: 1g; Protein: 15g; Total Carbs: 65g; Fiber: 15g; Sugar: 13g; Sodium: 540mg

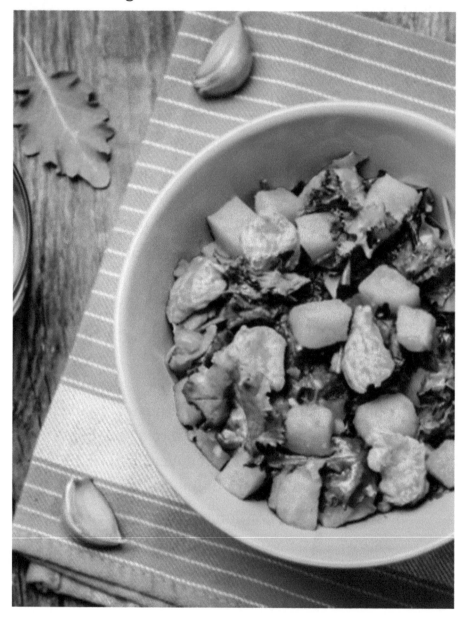

Slow Cooker Two-Bean Sloppy Joes

Preparation Time: 10 minutes

Cooking Time*: 6 hours*

Servings: *4*

Ingredients:

- 1 (15-ounce) can low-sodium black beans
- 1 (15-ounce) can low-sodium pinto beans
- 1 (15-ounce) can no-salt-added diced tomatoes
- 1 medium green bell pepper, cored, seeded, and chopped
- 1 medium yellow onion, chopped
- ¼ cup low-sodium vegetable broth
- 2 garlic cloves, minced
- 2 servings (¼ cup) meal prep barbecue sauce or bottled barbecue sauce
- ¼ teaspoon salt
- ¼ teaspoon freshly ground black pepper
- 4 whole-wheat buns

Directions:

1. In a slow cooker, combine the black beans, pinto beans, diced tomatoes, bell pepper, onion, broth, garlic, meal prep barbecue sauce, salt, and black pepper. Stir the **Ingredients** , then cover and cook on low for 6 hours.

2. Into each of 4 containers, spoon 1¼ cups of sloppy joe mix. Serve with 1 whole-wheat bun.

3. Storage: place airtight containers in the refrigerator for up to 1 week. To freeze, place freezer-safe containers in the freezer for up to 2 months. To defrost, refrigerate overnight. To reheat individual portions, microwave uncovered on high for 2 to 21/2 minutes. Alternatively, reheat the entire dish in a saucepan on the stove top. Bring the sloppy joes to a boil, then reduce the heat and simmer until heated through, 10 to 15 minutes. Serve with a whole-wheat bun.

Nutrition: Calories: 392; Total Fat: 3g; Saturated Fat: 0g; Protein: 17g; Total Carbs: 79g; Fiber: 19g; Sugar: 15g; Sodium: 759mg

Lighter Eggplant Parmesan

Preparation Time: 15 minutes

Cooking Time: 35 minutes

Servings: *4*

Ingredients:

- Nonstick cooking spray
- 3 eggs, beaten
- 1 tablespoon dried parsley
- 2 teaspoons ground oregano
- 1/8 teaspoon freshly ground black pepper
- 1 cup panko bread crumbs, preferably whole-wheat
- 1 large eggplant (about 2 pounds)
- 5 servings (21/2 cups) chunky tomato sauce or jarred low-sodium tomato sauce
- 1 cup part-skim mozzarella cheese
- ¼ cup grated parmesan cheese

Directions:

1. Preheat the oven to 450f. Coat a baking sheet with cooking spray.

2. In a medium bowl, whisk together the eggs, parsley, oregano, and pepper.

3. Pour the panko into a separate medium bowl.

4. Slice the eggplant into ¼-inch-thick slices. Dip each slice of eggplant into the egg mixture, shaking off the excess. Then dredge both sides of the eggplant in the panko bread crumbs. Place the coated eggplant on the prepared baking sheet, leaving a 1/2-inch space between each slice.

5. Bake for about 15 minutes until soft and golden brown. Remove from the oven and set aside to slightly cool.

6. Pour 1/2 cup of chunky tomato sauce on the bottom of an 8-by-15-inch baking dish. Using a spatula or the back of a spoon spread the tomato sauce evenly. Place half the slices of cooked eggplant, slightly overlapping, in the dish, and top with 1 cup of chunky tomato sauce, 1/2 cup of mozzarella and 2 tablespoons of grated parmesan. Repeat the layer, ending with the cheese.

7. Bake uncovered for 20 minutes until the cheese is bubbling and slightly browned.

8. Remove from the oven and allow cooling for 15 minutes before dividing the eggplant equally into 4 separate containers.

Nutrition: Calories: 333; Total Fat: 14g; Saturated Fat: 6g; Protein: 20g; Total Carbs: 35g; Fiber: 11g; Sugar: 15g; Sodium: 994mg

Coconut-Lentil Curry

Preparation Time: 15 minutes

Cooking Time: 35 minutes

Servings: *4*

Ingredients:

- 1 tablespoon olive oil
- 1 medium yellow onion, chopped
- 1 garlic clove, minced
- 1 medium red bell pepper, diced
- 1 (15-ounce) can green or brown lentils, rinsed and drained
- 2 medium sweet potatoes, washed, peeled, and cut into bite-size chunks (about 1¼ pounds)
- 1 (15-ounce) can no-salt-added diced tomatoes
- 2 tablespoons tomato paste
- 4 teaspoons curry powder
- 1/8 teaspoon ground cloves
- 1 (15-ounce) can light coconut milk
- ¼ teaspoon salt
- 2 pieces whole-wheat naan bread, halved, or 4 slices crusty bread

Directions:

1. In a large saucepan over medium heat, heat the olive oil. When the oil is shimmering, add both the onion and garlic and cook until the onion softens and the garlic is sweet, for about 3 minutes.

2. Add the bell pepper and continue cooking until it softens, about 5 minutes more. Add the lentils, sweet potatoes, tomatoes, tomato paste, curry powder, and cloves, and bring the mixture to a boil. Reduce the heat to medium-low, cover, and simmer until the potatoes are softened, about 20 minutes.

3. Add the coconut milk and salt, and return to a boil. Reduce the heat and simmer until the flavors combine, about 5 minutes.

4. Into each of 4 containers, spoon 2 cups of curry.

5. Enjoy each **Serving** with half of a piece of naan bread or 1 slice of crusty bread.

Nutrition: Calories: 559; Total Fat: 16g; Saturated Fat: 7g; Protein: 16g; Total Carbs: 86g; Fiber: 16g; Sugar: 18g; Sodium: 819mg

Stuffed Portobello with Cheese

Preparation Time: 15 minutes

Cooking Time: 25 minutes

Servings: *4*

Ingredients:

- 4 Portobello mushroom caps
- 1 tablespoon olive oil
- 1/2 teaspoon salt, divided
- ¼ teaspoon freshly ground black pepper, divided
- 1 cup baby spinach, chopped
- 11/2 cups part-skim ricotta cheese
- 1/2 cup part-skim shredded mozzarella cheese
- ¼ cup grated parmesan cheese
- 1 garlic clove, minced
- 1 tablespoon dried parsley
- 2 teaspoons dried oregano
- 4 teaspoons unseasoned bread crumbs, divided
- 4 servings (4 cups) roasted broccoli with shallots

Directions:

1. Preheat the oven to 375f. Line a baking sheet with aluminum foil.

2. Brush the mushroom caps with the olive oil, and sprinkle with ¼ teaspoon salt and 1/8 teaspoon pepper. Put the mushroom caps on the prepared baking sheet and bake until soft, about 12 minutes.

3. In a medium bowl, mix together the spinach, ricotta, mozzarella, parmesan, garlic, parsley, oregano, and the remaining ¼ teaspoon of salt and 1/8 teaspoon of pepper.

4. Spoon 1/2 cup of cheese mixture into each mushroom cap, and sprinkle each with 1 teaspoon of bread crumbs. Return the mushrooms to the oven for an additional 8 to 10 minutes until warmed through.

5. Remove from the oven and allow the mushrooms to cool for about 10 minutes before placing each in an individual container. Add 1 cup of roasted broccoli with shallots to each container.

Nutrition: Calories: 419; Total Fat: 30g; Saturated Fat: 10g; Protein: 23g; Total Carbs: 19g; Fiber: 2g; Sugar: 3g; Sodium: 790mg

Lighter Shrimp Scampi

Preparation Time: 15 minutes

Cooking Time: 15 minutes

Servings: *4*

Ingredients:

- 11/2 pounds large peeled and deveined shrimp
- ¼ teaspoon salt
- 1/8 teaspoon freshly ground black pepper
- 2 tablespoons olive oil
- 1 shallot, chopped
- 2 garlic cloves, minced
- ¼ cup cooking white wine
- Juice of 1/2 lemon (1 tablespoon)
- 1/2 teaspoon sriracha
- 2 tablespoons unsalted butter, at room temperature
- ¼ cup chopped fresh parsley
- 4 servings (6 cups) zucchini noodles with lemon vinaigrette

Directions:

1. Season the shrimp with the salt and pepper.

2. In a medium saucepan over medium heat, heat the oil. Add the shallot and garlic, and cook until the shallot softens and the garlic is fragrant, about 3 minutes. Add the shrimp, cover, and cook until opaque, 2 to 3 minutes on each side. Using a slotted spoon, transfer the shrimp to a large plate.

3. Add the wine, lemon juice, and sriracha to the saucepan, and stir to combine. Bring the mixture to a boil, then reduce the heat and simmer until the liquid is reduced by about half, 3 minutes. Add the butter and stir until melted, about 3 minutes. Return the shrimp to the saucepan and toss to coat. Add the parsley and stir to combine.

4. Into each of 4 containers, place 11/2 cups of zucchini noodles with lemon vinaigrette, and top with ¾ cup of scampi.

Nutrition: Calories: 364; Total Fat: 21g; Saturated Fat: 6g; Protein: 37g; Total Carbs: 10g; Fiber: 2g; Sugar: 6g; Sodium: 557mg

Maple-Mustard Salmon

Preparation Time: 10 minutes, plus 30 minutes marinating time

Cooking Time: 20 minutes

Servings: *4*

Ingredients:

- Nonstick cooking spray
- 1/2 cup 100% maple syrup
- 2 tablespoons Dijon mustard
- ¼ teaspoon salt
- 4 (5-ounce) salmon fillets
- 4 servings (4 cups) roasted broccoli with shallots
- 4 servings (2 cups) parleyed whole-wheat couscous

Directions:

1. Preheat the oven to 400f. Line a baking sheet with aluminum foil and coat with cooking spray.
2. In a medium bowl, whisk together the maple syrup, mustard, and salt until smooth.

3. Put the salmon fillets into the bowl and toss to coat. Cover and place in the refrigerator to marinate for at least 30 minutes and up to overnight.

4. Shake off excess marinade from the salmon fillets and place them on the prepared baking sheet, leaving a 1-inch space between each fillet. Discard the extra marinade.

5. Bake for about 20 minutes until the salmon is opaque and a thermometer inserted in the thickest part of a fillet reads 145f.

6. Into each of 4 resealable containers, place 1 salmon fillet, 1 cup of roasted broccoli with shallots, and 1/2 cup of parleyed whole-wheat couscous.

Nutrition: Calories: 601; Total Fat: 29g; Saturated Fat: 4g; Protein: 36g; Total Carbs: 51g; Fiber: 3g; Sugar: 23g; Sodium: 610mg

Chicken Salad with Grapes and Pecans

Preparation Time: 15 Minutes

Cooking Time: 5 Minutes

Servings: *4*

Ingredients:

- 1/3 cup unsalted pecans, chopped
- 10 ounces cooked skinless, boneless chicken breast or rotisserie chicken, finely chopped
- 1/2 medium yellow onion, finely chopped
- 1 celery stalk, finely chopped
- ¾ cup red or green seedless grapes, halved
- ¼ cup light mayonnaise
- ¼ cup nonfat plain Greek yogurt
- 1 tablespoon Dijon mustard
- 1 tablespoon dried parsley
- ¼ teaspoon salt
- 1/8 teaspoon freshly ground black pepper
- 1 cup shredded romaine lettuce
- 4 (8-inch) whole-wheat pitas

Directions:

1. Heat a small skillet over medium-low heat to toast the pecans. Cook the pecans until fragrant, about 3 minutes. Remove from the heat and set aside to cool.

2. In a medium bowl, mix the chicken, onion, celery, pecans, and grapes.

3. In a small bowl, whisk together the mayonnaise, yogurt, mustard, parsley, salt, and pepper. Spoon the sauce over the chicken mixture and stir until well combined.

4. Into each of 4 containers, place ¼ cup of lettuce and top with 1 cup of chicken salad. Store the pitas separately until ready to serve.

5. When ready to eat, stuff the **Serving** of salad and lettuce into 1 pita.

Nutrition: Calories: 418; Total Fat: 14g; Saturated Fat: 2g; Protein: 31g; Total Carbs: 43g; Fiber: 6g;

Roasted Vegetables

Preparation Time: 14 minutes

Cooking Time: 17 minutes

Servings: *3*

Ingredients:

- 4 Tbsp. olive oil, reserve some for greasing
- 2 heads, large garlic, tops sliced off
- 2 large eggplants/aubergine, tops removed, cubed
- 2 large shallots, peeled, quartered
- 1 large carrot, peeled, cubed
- 1 large parsnips, peeled, cubed
- 1 small green bell pepper, deseeded, ribbed, cubed
- 1 small red bell pepper, deseeded, ribbed, cubed
- ½ pound Brussels sprouts, halved, do not remove cores
- 1 sprig, large thyme, leaves picked
- sea salt, coarse-grained

For garnish

- 1 large lemon, halved, ½ squeezed, ½ sliced into smaller wedges
- 1/8 cup fennel bulb, minced

Directions:

1. From 425°F or 220°C preheat oven for at least 5 minutes before using.

2. Line deep roasting pan with aluminum foil; lightly grease with oil. Tumble in bell peppers, Brussels sprouts, carrots, eggplants, garlic, parsnips, rosemary leaves, shallots, and thyme. Add a pinch of sea salt; drizzle in remaining oil and lemon juice. Toss well to combine.

3. Cover roasting pan with a sheet of aluminum foil. Place this on middle rack of oven. Bake for 20 to 30 minutes. Remove aluminum foil. Roast, for another 5 to 10 minutes, or until some vegetables brown at the edges. Remove roasting pan from oven. Cool slightly before ladling equal portions into plates.

4. Garnish with fennel and a wedge of lemon. Squeeze lemon juice on top of dish before eating.

Nutrition: Calories 163; Total Fat 4.2 g; Saturated Fat 0.8 g; Cholesterol 0 mg; Sodium 861 mg; Total Carbs 22.5 g; Fiber 6.3 g; Sugar 2.3 g; Protein 9.2 g

Millet Pilaf

Preparation Time: 10 minutes

Cooking Time: *15 minutes*

Servings: *4*

Ingredients:

- 1 cup millet
- 2 tomatoes, rinsed, seeded, and chopped
- 1¾ cups filtered water
- 2 tablespoons extra-virgin olive oil
- ¼ cup chopped dried apricot
- Zest of 1 lemon
- Juice of 1 lemon
- ½ cup fresh parsley, rinsed and chopped
- Himalayan pink salt
- Freshly ground black pepper

Directions:

1. In an electric pressure cooker, combine the millet, tomatoes, and water. Lock the lid into place, select Manual and High Pressure, and cook for 7 minutes.

2. When the beep sounds, quick release the pressure by pressing Cancel and twisting the

steam valve to the Venting position. Carefully remove the lid.

3. Stir in the olive oil, apricot, lemon zest, lemon juice, and parsley. Taste, season with salt and pepper, and serve.

_Nutrition__:_ Calories: 270; Total fat: 8g; Total carbohydrates: 42g; Fiber: 5g; Sugar: 3g; Protein: 6g

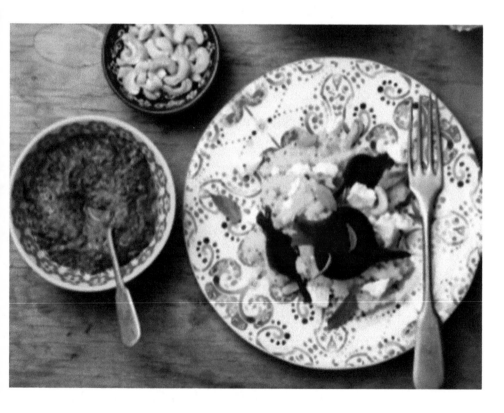

Sweet and Sour Onions

Preparation Time: 10 minutes

Cooking Time: 11 minutes

Servings: *4*

Ingredients:

- 4 large onions, halved
- 2 garlic cloves, crushed
- 3 cups vegetable stock
- 1 ½ tablespoon balsamic vinegar
- ½ teaspoon Dijon mustard
- 1 tablespoon sugar

Directions:

1. Combine onions and garlic in a pan. Fry for 3 minutes, or till softened.
2. Pour stock, vinegar, Dijon mustard, and sugar. Bring to a boil.
3. Reduce heat. Cover and let the combination simmer for 10 minutes.
4. Get rid of from heat. Continue stirring until the liquid is reduced and the onions are brown. Serve.

Nutrition: Calories 203; Total Fat 41.2 g; Saturated Fat 0.8 g; Cholesterol 0 mg; Sodium 861 mg; Total Carbs 29.5 g; Fiber 16.3 g; Sugar 29.3 g; Protein 19.2 g

Sautéed Apples and Onions

Preparation Time: 14 minutes

Cooking Time: 16 minutes

Servings: _3_

Ingredients:

- 2 cups dry cider
- 1 large onion, halved
- 2 cups vegetable stock
- 4 apples, sliced into wedges
- Pinch of salt
- Pinch of pepper

Directions:

1. Combine cider and onion in a saucepan. Bring to a boil until the onions are cooked and liquid almost gone.

2. Pour the stock and the apples. Season with salt and pepper. Stir occasionally. Cook for about 10 minutes or until the apples are tender but not mushy. Serve.

Nutrition: Calories 343; Total Fat 51.2 g; Saturated Fat 0.8 g; Cholesterol 0 mg; Sodium 861 mg; Total Carbs 22.5 g; Fiber 6.3 g; Sugar 2.3 g; Protein 9.2 g

Zucchini Noodles with Portabella Mushrooms

Preparation Time: 14 minutes

Cooking Time: 16 minutes

Servings: *3*

Ingredients:

- 1 zucchini, processed into spaghetti-like noodles
- 3 garlic cloves, minced
- 2 white onions, thinly sliced
- 1 thumb-sized ginger, julienned
- 1 lb. chicken thighs
- 1 lb. portabella mushrooms, sliced into thick slivers
- 2 cups chicken stock
- 3 cups water
- Pinch of sea salt, add more if needed
- Pinch of black pepper, add more if needed
- 2 tsp. sesame oil
- 4 Tbsp. coconut oil, divided
- ¼ cup fresh chives, minced, for garnish

Directions:

1. Pour 2 tablespoons of coconut oil into a large saucepan. Fry mushroom slivers in batches for 5 minutes or until seared brown. Set aside. Transfer these to a plate.

2. Sauté the onion, garlic, and ginger for 3 minutes or until tender. Add in chicken thighs, cooked mushrooms, chicken stock, water, salt, and pepper stir mixture well. Bring to a boil.

3. Decrease gradually the heat and allow simmering for 20 minutes or until the chicken is forking tender. Tip in sesame oil.

4. Serve by placing an equal amount of zucchini noodles into bowls. Ladle soup and garnish with chives.

Nutrition: Calories 163; Total Fat 4.2 g; Saturated Fat 0.8 g; Cholesterol 0 mg; Sodium 861 mg; Total Carbs 22.5 g; Fiber 6.3 g; Sugar 2.3 g; Protein 9.2 g

Grilled Tempeh with Pineapple

Preparation Time: 12 minutes

Cooking Time: 16 minutes

Servings: *3*

Ingredients:

- 10 oz. tempeh, sliced
- 1 red bell pepper, quartered
- 1/4 pineapple, sliced into rings
- 6 oz. green beans
- 1 tbsp. coconut aminos
- 2 1/2 tbsp. orange juice, freshly squeeze
- 1 1/2 tbsp. lemon juice, freshly squeezed
- 1 tbsp. extra virgin olive oil
- 1/4 cup hoisin sauce

Directions:

1. Blend together the olive oil, orange and lemon juices, coconut aminos or soy sauce, and hoisin sauce in a bowl. Add the diced tempeh and set aside.

2. Heat up the grill or place a grill pan over medium high flame. Once hot, lift the marinated tempeh from the bowl with a pair of tongs and transfer them to the grill or pan.

3. Grille for 2 to 3 minutes, or until browned all over.

4. Grill the sliced pineapples alongside the tempeh, then transfer them directly onto the **Serving** platter.

5. Place the grilled tempeh beside the grilled pineapple and cover with aluminum foil to keep warm.

6. Meanwhile, place the green beans and bell peppers in a bowl and add just enough of the marinade to coat.

7. Prepare the grill pan and add the vegetables. Grill until fork tender and slightly charred.

8. Transfer the grilled vegetables to the **Serving** platter and arrange artfully with the tempeh and pineapple. Serve at once.

Nutrition: Calories 163; Total Fat 4.2 g; Saturated Fat 0.8 g; Cholesterol 0 mg; Sodium 861 mg; Total Carbs 22.5 g; Fiber 6.3 g; Sugar 2.3 g; Protein 9.2 g

Courgettes In Cider Sauce

Preparation Time: 13 minutes

Cooking Time: 17 minutes

Servings: _3_

Ingredients:

- 2 cups baby courgettes
- 3 tablespoons vegetable stock
- 2 tablespoons apple cider vinegar
- 1 tablespoon light brown sugar
- 4 spring onions, finely sliced
- 1-piece fresh gingerroot, grated
- 1 teaspoon corn flour
- 2 teaspoons water

Directions:

1. Bring a pan with salted water to a boil. Add courgettes. Bring to a boil for 5 minutes.
2. Meanwhile, in a pan, combine vegetable stock, apple cider vinegar, brown sugar, onions, gingerroot, lemon juice and rind, and orange juice and rind. Take to a boil. Lower the heat and allow simmering for 3 minutes.

3. Mix the corn flour with water. Stir well. Pour into the sauce. Continue stirring until the sauce thickens.

4. Drain courgettes. Transfer to the **Serving** dish. Spoon over the sauce. Toss to coat courgettes. Serve.

Nutrition: Calories 173; Total Fat 9.2 g; Saturated Fat 0.8 g; Cholesterol 0 mg; Sodium 861 mg; Total Carbs 22.5 g; Fiber 6.3 g; Sugar 2.3 g; Protein 9.2 g

Baked Mixed Mushrooms

Preparation Time: 8 minutes

Cooking Time: 20 minutes

Servings: *3*

Ingredients:

- 2 cups mixed wild mushrooms
- 1 cup chestnut mushrooms
- 2 cups dried porcini
- 2 shallots
- 4 garlic cloves
- 3 cups raw pecans
- ½ bunch fresh thyme
- 1 bunch flat-leaf parsley
- 2 tablespoons olive oil
- 2 fresh bay leaves
- 1 ½ cups stale bread

Directions:

1. Remove skin and finely chop garlic and shallots. Roughly chop the wild mushrooms and chestnut mushrooms. Pick the leaves of the

thyme and tear the bread into small pieces. Put inside the pressure cooker.

2. Place the pecans and roughly chop the nuts. Pick the parsley leaves and roughly chop.

3. Place the porcini in a bowl then add 300ml of boiling water. Set aside until needed.

4. Heat oil in the pressure cooker. Add the garlic and shallots. Cook for 3 minutes while stirring occasionally.

5. Drain porcini and reserve the liquid. Add the porcini into the pressure cooker together with the wild mushrooms and chestnut mushrooms. Add the bay leaves and thyme.

6. Position the lid and lock in place. Put to high heat and bring to high pressure. Adjust heat to stabilize. Cook for 10 minutes. Adjust taste if necessary.

7. Transfer the mushroom mixture into a bowl and set aside to cool completely.

8. Once the mushrooms are completely cool, add the bread, pecans, a pinch of black pepper and sea salt, and half of the reserved liquid into the bowl. Mix well. Add more reserved liquid if the mixture seems dry.

9. Add more than half of the parsley into the bowl and stir. Transfer the mixture into a 20cm x

25cm lightly greased baking dish and cover with tin foil.

10.   Bake in the oven for 35 minutes. Then, get rid of the foil and cook for another 10 minutes. Once done, sprinkle the remaining parsley on top and serve with bread or crackers. Serve.

Nutrition: Calories 343; Total Fat 4.2 g; Saturated Fat 0.8 g; Cholesterol 0 mg; Sodium 861 mg; Total Carbs 22.5 g; Fiber 6.3 g; Sugar 2.3 g; Protein 9.2 g

Spiced Okra

Preparation Time: 14 minutes

Cooking Time: 16 minutes

Servings: *3*

Ingredients:

- 2 cups okra
- ¼ teaspoon stevia
- 1 teaspoon chilli powder
- ½ teaspoon ground turmeric
- 1 tablespoon ground coriander
- 2 tablespoons fresh coriander, chopped
- 1 tablespoon ground cumin
- ¼ teaspoon salt
- 1 tablespoon desiccated coconut
- 3 tablespoons vegetable oil
- ½ teaspoon black mustard seeds
- ½ teaspoon cumin seeds
- Fresh tomatoes, to garnish

Directions:

1. Trim okra. Wash and dry.

2. Combine stevia, chilli powder, turmeric, ground coriander, fresh coriander, cumin, salt, and desiccated coconut in a bowl.

3. Heat the oil in a pan. Cook mustard and cumin seeds for 3 minutes. Stir continuously. Add okra. Tip in the spice mixture. Cook on low heat for 8 minutes.

4. Transfer to a **Serving** dish. Garnish with fresh tomatoes.

__Nutrition:__ Calories 163; Total Fat 4.2 g; Saturated Fat 0.8 g; Cholesterol 0 mg; Sodium 861 mg; Total Carbs 22.5 g; Fiber 6.3 g; Sugar 2.3 g; Protein 9.2 g

Lemony Salmon Burgers

Preparation Time: *10 Minutes*

Cooking Time: 10 Minutes

Servings: *4*

Ingredients:

- 2 (3-oz) cans boneless, skinless pink salmon
- 1/4 cup panko breadcrumbs
- 4 tsp. lemon juice
- 1/4 cup red bell pepper
- 1/4 cup sugar-free yogurt
- 1 egg
- 2 (1.5-oz) whole wheat hamburger toasted buns

Directions:

1. Mix drained and flaked salmon, finely-chopped bell pepper, panko breadcrumbs.
2. Combine 2 tbsp. cup sugar-free yogurt, 3 tsp. fresh lemon juice, and egg in a bowl. Shape mixture into 2 (3-inch) patties, bake on the skillet over medium heat 4 to 5 Minutes per side.

3. Stir together 2 tbsp. sugar-free yogurt and 1 tsp. lemon juice; spread over bottom halves of buns.

4. Top each with 1 patty, and cover with bun tops.

This dish is very mouth-watering!

Nutrition: Calories 131; Protein 12; Fat 1 g; Carbs 19 g

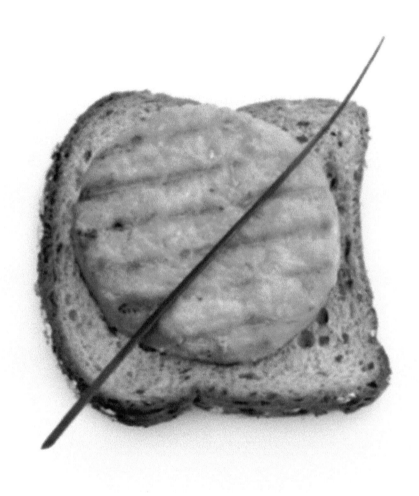

Caprese Turkey Burgers

Preparation Time: *10 Minutes*
Cooking Time: 10 Minutes
Servings: *4*

Ingredients:

- 1/2 lb. 93% lean ground turkey
- 2 (1,5-oz) whole wheat hamburger buns (toasted)
- 1/4 cup shredded mozzarella cheese (part-skim) `
- 1 egg
- 1 big tomato
- 1 small clove garlic
- 4 large basil leaves
- 1/8 tsp. salt
- 1/8 tsp. pepper

Directions:

1. Combine turkey, white egg, Minced garlic, salt, and pepper (mix until combined);

2. Shape into 2 cutlets. Put cutlets into a skillet; cook 5 to 7 Minutes per side.

3. Top cutlets properly with cheese and sliced tomato at the end of cooking.

4. Put 1 cutlet on the bottom of each bun.

5. Top each patty with 2 basil leaves. Cover with bun tops.

My guests enjoy this dish every time they visit my home.

Nutrition: Calories 180; Protein 7 g; Fat 4 g; Carbs 20 g

Pasta Salad

Preparation Time: *15 Minutes*

Cooking Time: 15 Minutes

Servings: *4*

Ingredients:

- 8 oz. whole-wheat pasta
- 2 tomatoes
- 1 (5-oz) pkg spring mix
- 9 slices bacon
- 1/3 cup mayonnaise (reduced-fat)
- 1 tbsp. Dijon mustard
- 3 tbsp. apple cider vinegar
- 1/4 tsp. salt
- 1/2 tsp. pepper

Directions:

1. Cook pasta.
2. Chilled pasta, chopped tomatoes and spring mix in a bowl.
3. Crumble cooked bacon over pasta.

4. Combine mayonnaise, mustard, vinegar, salt and pepper in a small bowl.

5. Pour dressing over pasta, stirring to coat.

Understanding diabetes is the first step in curing.

Nutrition: Calories 200; Protein 15 g; Fat 3 g; Carbs 6 g

Chicken, Strawberry, And Avocado Salad

Preparation Time: *10 Minutes*

Cooking Time: 5 Minutes

Ingredients:

- 1,5 cups chicken (skin removed)
- 1/4 cup almonds
- 2 (5-oz) pkg salad greens
- 1 (16-oz) pkg strawberries
- 1 avocado
- 1/4 cup green onion
- 1/4 cup lime juice
- 3 tbsp. extra virgin olive oil
- 2 tbsp. honey
- 1/4 tsp. salt
- 1/4 tsp. pepper

Directions:

1. Toast almonds until golden and fragrant.
2. Mix lime juice, oil, honey, salt, and pepper.

3. Mix greens, sliced strawberries, chicken, diced avocado, and sliced green onion and sliced almonds; drizzle with dressing. Toss to coat.

Yummy!

Nutrition: Calories 150;Protein 15 g; Fat 10 g; Carbs 5 g

Lemon-Thyme Eggs

Preparation Time: 10 Minutes

Cooking Time: 5 Minutes

Servings: *4*

Ingredients:

- 7 large eggs
- 1/4 cup mayonnaise (reduced-fat)
- 2 tsp. lemon juice
- 1 tsp. Dijon mustard
- 1 tsp. chopped fresh thyme
- 1/8 tsp. cayenne pepper

Directions:

1. Bring eggs to a boil.
2. Peel and cut each egg in half lengthwise.
3. Remove yolks to a bowl. Add mayonnaise, lemon juice, mustard, thyme, and cayenne to egg yolks; mash to blend. Fill egg white halves with yolk mixture.
4. Chill until ready to serve.

Please your family with a delicious meal.

_Nutrition__:_ Calories 40; Protein 10 g; Fat 6 g; Carbs 2 g

Spinach Salad with Bacon

Preparation Time: *15 Minutes*

Cooking Time: 0 Minutes

Servings: *4*

Ingredients:

- 8 slices center-cut bacon
- 3 tbsp. extra virgin olive oil
- 1 (5-oz) pkg baby spinach
- 1 tbsp. apple cider vinegar
- 1 tsp. Dijon mustard
- 1/2 tsp. honey
- 1/4 tsp. salt
- 1/2 tsp. pepper

Directions:

1. Mix vinegar, mustard, honey, salt and pepper in a bowl.
2. Whisk in oil. Place spinach in a **Serving** bowl; drizzle with dressing, and toss to coat.
3. Sprinkle with cooked and crumbled bacon.
4.

Nutrition: Calories 110; Protein 6 g; Fat 2 g; Carbs 1 g

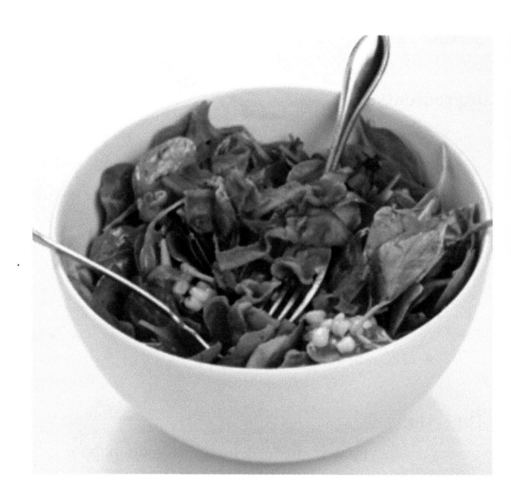

Pea and Collards Soup

Preparation Time: *10 Minutes*

Cooking Time: 50 Minutes

Servings: *4*

Ingredients:

- 1/2 (16-oz) pkg black-eyed peas
- 1 onion
- 2 carrots
- 1,5 cups ham (low-sodium)
- 1 (1-lb) bunch collard greens (trimmed)
- 1 tbsp. extra virgin olive oil
- 2 cloves garlic
- 1/2 tsp. black pepper
- Hot sauce

Directions:

1. Cook chopped onion and carrots 10 Minutes.
2. Add peas, diced ham, collards, and Minced garlic. Cook 5 Minutes.

3. Add broth, 3 cups water, and pepper. Bring to a boil; simmer 35 Minutes, adding water if needed.

Serve with favorite sauce.

Nutrition: Calories 86; Protein 15 g; Fat 2 g; Carbs 9 g

Spanish Stew

Preparation Time: *10 Minutes*

Cooking Time: 25 Minutes

Servings: *4*

Ingredients:

- 1.1/2 (12-oz) pkg smoked chicken sausage links
- 1 (5-oz) pkg baby spinach
- 1 (15-oz) can chickpeas
- 1 (14.5-oz) can tomatoes with basil, garlic, and oregano
- 1/2 tsp. smoked paprika
- 1/2 tsp. cumin
- 3/4 cup onions
- 1 tbsp. extra virgin olive oil

Directions:

1. Cook sliced the sausage in hot oil until browned. Remove from pot.
2. Add chopped onions; cook until tender.

3. Add sausage, drained and rinsed chickpeas, diced tomatoes, paprika, and ground cumin. Cook 15 Minutes.

4. Add in spinach; cook 1 to 2 Minutes.

This dish is ideal for every day and for a festive table.

Nutrition: Calories 200; Protein 10 g; Fat 20 g; Carbs 1 g

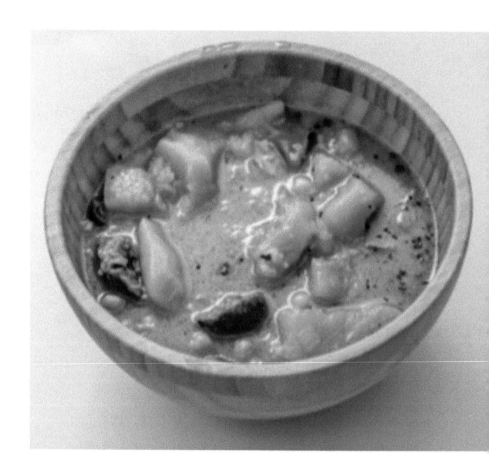

Creamy Taco Soup

Preparation Time: 10 Minutes

Cooking Time: 20 Minutes

Servings: *4*

Ingredients:

- 3/4 lb. ground sirloin
- 1/2 (8-oz) cream cheese
- 1/2 onion
- 1 clove garlic
- 1 (10-oz) can tomatoes and green chiles
- 1 (14.5-oz) can beef broth
- 1/4 cup heavy cream
- 1,5 tsp. cumin
- 1/2 tsp. chili powder

Directions:

1. Cook beef, chopped onion, and Minced garlic until meat is browned and crumbly; drain and return to pot.

2. Add ground cumin, chili powder, and cream cheese cut into small pieces and softened, stirring until cheese is melted.

3. Add diced tomatoes, broth, and cream; bring to a boil, and simmer 10 Minutes. Season with pepper and salt to taste.

You've got to give someone the recipe for this soup dish!

Nutrition: Calories 60; Protein 3 g; Fat 1 g; Carbs 8 g

Chicken with Caprese Salsa

Preparation Time: *15 Minutes*

Cooking Time: 5 Minutes

Servings: *4*

Ingredients:

- 3/4 lb. boneless, skinless chicken breasts
- 2 big tomatoes
- 1/2 (8-oz) ball fresh mozzarella cheese
- 1/4 cup red onion
- 2 tbsp. fresh basil
- 1 tbsp. balsamic vinegar
- 2 tbsp. extra virgin olive oil (divided)
- 1/2 tsp. salt (divided)
- 1/4 tsp. pepper (divided)

Directions:

1. Sprinkle cut in half lengthwise chicken with 1/4 tsp. salt and 1/8 tsp. pepper.
2. Heat 1 tbsp. olive oil, cook chicken 5 Minutes.
3. Meanwhile, mix chopped tomatoes, diced cheese, finely chopped onion, chopped basil,

vinegar, 1 tbsp. oil, and 1/4 tsp. salt and 1/8 tsp. pepper.

4. Spoon salsa over chicken.

Chicken with Caprese Salsa is a nutritious, simple and very tasty dish that can be prepared in a few Minutes.

Nutrition: Calories 210; Protein 28 g; Fat 17 g; Carbs 0, 1 g

Balsamic-Roasted Broccoli

Preparation Time: *10 Minutes*
Cooking Time: 15 Minutes
Servings: *4*

Ingredients:

- 1 lb. broccoli
- 1 tbsp. extra virgin olive oil
- 1 tbsp. balsamic vinegar
- 1 clove garlic
- 1/8 tsp. salt
- Pepper to taste

Directions:

1. Preheat oven to 450F.
2. Combine broccoli, olive oil, vinegar, Minced garlic, salt, and pepper; toss.
3. Spread broccoli on a baking sheet.
4. Bake 12 to 15 Minutes.

Really good!

Nutrition: Calories 27; Protein 3 g; Fat 0, 3 g; Carbs 4 g

Hearty Beef and Vegetable Soup

Preparation Time: *10 Minutes*

Cooking Time: 30 Minutes

Servings: *4*

Ingredients:

- 1/2 lb. lean ground beef
- 2 cups beef broth
- 1,5 tbsp. vegetable oil (divided)
- 1 cup green bell pepper
- 1/2 cup red onion
- 1 cup green cabbage
- 1 cup frozen mixed vegetables
- 1/2 can tomatoes
- 1,5 tsp. Worcestershire sauce
- 1 small bay leaf
- 1,8 tsp. pepper
- 2 tbsp. ketchup

Directions:

1. Cook beef in 1/2 tbsp. hot oil 2 Minutes.

2. Stir in chopped bell pepper and chopped onion; cook 4 Minutes.

3. Add chopped cabbage, mixed vegetables, stewed tomatoes, broth, Worcestershire sauce, bay leaf, and pepper; bring to a boil.

4. Reduce heat to medium; cover, and cook 15 Minutes.

5. Stir in ketchup and 1 tbsp. oil, and remove from heat. Let stand 10 Minutes.

The right diet is excellent diabetes remedy.

Nutrition: Calories 170; Protein 17 g; Fat 8 g; Carbs 3 g

Cauliflower Muffin

Preparation Time: *15 Minutes*
Cooking Time: *30 Minutes*
Servings: *4*

Ingredients:

- 2,5 cup cauliflower
- 2/3 cup ham
- 2,5 cups of cheese
- 2/3 cup champignon
- 1,5 tbsp. flaxseed
- 3 eggs
- 1/4 tsp. salt
- 1/8 tsp. pepper

Directions:

1. 1. Preheat oven to 375 F.
2. Put muffin liners in a 12-muffin tin.
3. Combine diced cauliflower, ground flaxseed, beaten eggs, cup diced ham, grated cheese, and diced mushrooms, salt, pepper.
4. Divide mixture rightly between muffin liners.

5. Bake 30 Minutes.

This is a great lunch for the whole family.

Nutrition: Calories 116; Protein 10 g; Fat 7 g; Carbs 3 g

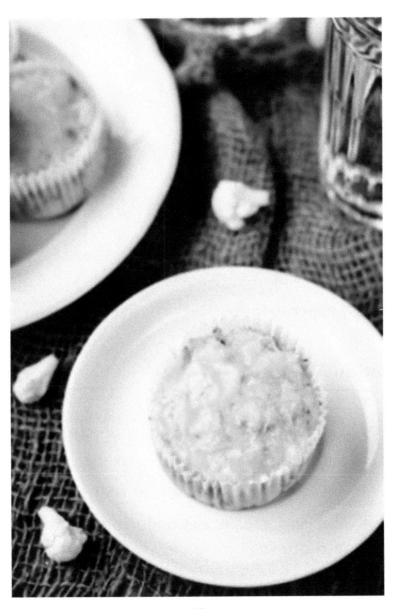

Ham and Egg Cups

Preparation Time: *10 Minutes*

Cooking Time: 15 Minutes

Servings: *4*

Ingredients:

- 5 slices ham
- 4 tbsp. cheese
- 1,5 tbsp. cream
- 3 egg whites
- 1,5 tbsp. pepper (green)
- 1 tsp. salt
- pepper to taste

Directions:

1. Preheat oven to 350 F.
2. Arrange each slice of thinly sliced ham into 4 muffin tin.
3. Put 1/4 of grated cheese into ham cup.
4. Mix eggs, cream, salt and pepper and divide it into 2 tins.

5. Bake in oven 15 Minutes; after baking, sprinkle with green onions.

If you want to keep your current shape, also pay attention to this dish.

__Nutrition__: Calories 180; Protein 13 g; Fat 13 g; Carbs 2 g

Lemony Salmon

Preparation Time: 10 minutes
Cooking Time: 3 Minutes
Servings: *3*

Ingredients:

- 1 pound salmon fillet, cut into 3 pieces
- 3 teaspoons fresh dill, chopped
- 5 tablespoons fresh lemon juice, divided
- Salt and ground black pepper, as required

Directions:

1. Arrange a steamer trivet in Instant Pot and pour ¼ cup of lemon juice.
2. Season the salmon with salt and black pepper evenly.
3. Place the salmon pieces on top of trivet, skin side down and drizzle with remaining lemon juice.
4. Now, sprinkle the salmon pieces with dill evenly.
5. Close the lid and place the pressure valve to "Seal" position.

6. Press "Steam" and use the default time of 3 minutes.

7. Press "Cancel" and allow a "Natural" release.

8. Open the lid and serve hot.

Nutrition: Calories: 20; Fats: 9.6g; Carbs: 1.1g; Sugar: 0.5g; Proteins: 29.7g; Sodium: 74mg

Shrimp with Green Beans

Preparation Time: 10 minutes

Cooking Time: 2 Minutes

Servings: *4*

Ingredients:

- ¾ pound fresh green beans, trimmed
- 1-pound medium frozen shrimp, peeled and deveined
- 2 tablespoons fresh lemon juice
- 2 tablespoons olive oil
- Salt and ground black pepper, as required

Directions:

1. Arrange a steamer trivet in the Instant Pot and pour cup of water.
2. Arrange the green beans on top of trivet in a single layer and top with shrimp.
3. Drizzle with oil and lemon juice.
4. Sprinkle with salt and black pepper.
5. Close the lid and place the pressure valve to "Seal" position.

6. Press "Steam" and just use the default time of 2 minutes.

7. Press "Cancel" and allow a "Natural" release.

8. Open the lid and serve.

Nutrition: Calories: 223; Fats: 1g; Carbs: 7.9g; Sugar: 1.4g; Proteins: 27.4g; Sodium: 322mg

Crab Curry

Preparation Time: 10 minutes

Cooking Time: 20 Minutes

Servings: *2*

Ingredients:

- 0.5lb chopped crab
- 1 thinly sliced red onion
- 0.5 cup chopped tomato
- 3tbsp curry paste
- 1tbsp oil or ghee

Directions:

1. Set the Instant Pot to sauté and add the onion, oil, and curry paste.
2. When the onion is soft, add the remaining Ingredients and seal.
3. Cook on Stew for 20 minutes.
4. Release the pressure naturally.

Nutrition: Calories: 2; Carbs: 11; Sugar: 4; Fat: 10; Protein: 24; GL: 9

Mixed Chowder

Preparation Time: 10 minutes

Cooking Time: 35 Minutes

Servings: *2*

Ingredients:

- 1lb fish stew mix
- 2 cups white sauce
- 3tbsp old bay seasoning

Directions:

1. Mix all the Ingredients in your Instant Pot.
2. Cook on Stew for 35 minutes.
3. Release the pressure naturally.

Nutrition: Calories: 320; Carbs: 9; Sugar: 2; Fat: 16; Protein: GL: 4

Mussels in Tomato Sauce

Preparation Time: 10 minutes

Cooking Time: 3 Minutes

Servings: *4*

Ingredients:

- 2 tomatoes, seeded and chopped finely
- 2 pounds mussels, scrubbed and de-bearded
- 1 cup low-sodium chicken broth
- 1 tablespoon fresh lemon juice
- 2 garlic cloves, minced

Directions:

1. In the pot of Instant Pot, place tomatoes, garlic, wine and bay leaf and stir to combine.
2. Arrange the mussels on top.
3. Close the lid and place the pressure valve to "Seal" position.
4. Press "Manual" and cook under "High Pressure" for about 3 minutes.
5. Press "Cancel" and carefully allow a "Quick" release.

6. Open the lid and serve hot.

Nutrition: Calories: 213; Fats: 25.2g; Carbs: 11g; Sugar: 1; Proteins: 28.2g; Sodium: 670mg

Citrus Salmon

Preparation Time: 10 minutes

Cooking Time: 7 Minutes

Servings: *4*

Ingredients:

- 4 (4-ounce) salmon fillets
- 1 cup low-sodium chicken broth
- 1 teaspoon fresh ginger, minced
- 2 teaspoons fresh orange zest, grated finely
- 3 tablespoons fresh orange juice
- 1 tablespoon olive oil
- Ground black pepper, as required

Directions:

1. In Instant Pot, add all Ingredients and mix.
2. Close the lid and place the pressure valve to "Seal" position.
3. Press "Manual" and cook under "High Pressure" for about 7 minutes.
4. Press "Cancel" and allow a "Natural" release.

5. Open the lid and serve the salmon fillets with the topping of cooking sauce.

Nutrition: Calories: 190; Fats: 10.5g; Carbs: 1.8g; Sugar: 1g; Proteins: 22. Sodium: 68mg

Herbed Salmon

Preparation Time: 10 minutes

Cooking Time: 3 Minutes

Servings: *4*

Ingredients:

- 4 (4-ounce) salmon fillets
- ¼ cup olive oil
- 2 tablespoons fresh lemon juice
- 1 garlic clove, minced
- ¼ teaspoon dried oregano
- Salt and ground black pepper, as required
- 4 fresh rosemary sprigs
- 4 lemon slices

Directions:

1. For dressing: in a large bowl, add oil, lemon juice, garlic, oregano, salt and black pepper and beat until well co combined.
2. Arrange a steamer trivet in the Instant Pot and pour 11/2 cups of water in Instant Pot.

3. Place the salmon fillets on top of trivet in a single layer and top with dressing.

4. Arrange 1 rosemary sprig and 1 lemon slice over each fillet.

5. Close the lid and place the pressure valve to "Seal" position.

6. Press "Steam" and just use the default time of 3 minutes.

7. Press "Cancel" and carefully allow a "Quick" release.

8. Open the lid and serve hot.

Nutrition: Calories: 262; Fats: 17g; Carbs: 0.7g; Sugar: 0.2g; Proteins: 22.1g; Sodium: 91mg

Salmon in Green Sauce

Preparation Time: 10 minutes

Cooking Time: 12 Minutes

Servings: *4*

Ingredients:

- 4 (6-ounce) salmon fillets
- 1 avocado, peeled, pitted and chopped
- 1/2 cup fresh basil, chopped
- 3 garlic cloves, chopped
- 1 tablespoon fresh lemon zest, grated finely

Directions:

1. Grease a large piece of foil.
2. In a large bowl, add all Ingredients except salmon and water and with a fork, mash completely.
3. Place fillets in the center of foil and top with avocado mixture evenly.
4. Fold the foil around fillets to seal them.
5. Arrange a steamer trivet in the Instant Pot and pour 1/2 cup of water.

6. Place the foil packet on top of trivet.

7. Close the lid and place the pressure valve to "Seal" position.

8. Press "Manual" and cook under "High Pressure" for about minutes.

9. Meanwhile, preheat the oven to broiler.

10. Press "Cancel" and allow a "Natural" release.

11. Open the lid and transfer the salmon fillets onto a broiler pan.

12. Broil for about 3-4 minutes.

13. Serve warm.

Nutrition: Calories: 333; Fats: 20.3g; Carbs: 5.5g; Sugar: 0.4g; Proteins; 34.2g; Sodium: 79mg

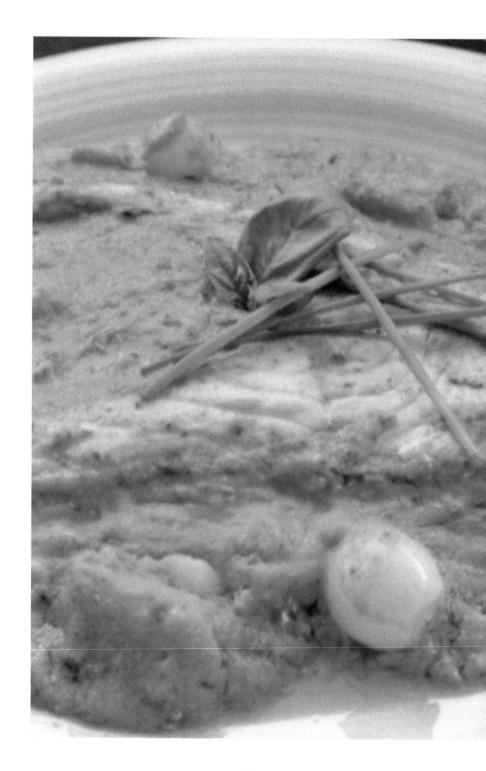

Lightning Source UK Ltd.
Milton Keynes UK
UKHW020645100621
385263UK00001B/141